TESTIMONIALS

Reading this book and taking it in can heal you in the deepest places where you didn't receive the love you needed. After 35 years supporting clients through dark nights of the soul, Beth and Margie have extraordinary insight into the tender, vulnerable, often hidden shards of brokenness we carry with us throughout our lives. This book is an outpouring of love so immense it can reach you in those places where you ache for someone to hold you with unconditional embrace. Few of us have ever felt absolute security and wholeness inside of us. This is Beth and Margie's heart felt blessing for us: to re-discover our birthrights as perfect beings of light and to find our way home.

~Erica Ariel Fox
New York Times bestselling author of
Winning From Within: A Breakthrough Method for Leading, Living, and Lasting Change

These profound messages go to the heart of the foundation of love—love and acceptance of self. The Secret To Loving Yourself is delicious food for the hungry heart. Thank you Beth and Margie.

~Richard Matzkin
author of *Loving Promises: The Master Class for Creating Magnificent Relationship*

The Secret to Loving Yourself is a wonderful, refined companion on the inner journey from shame to healthy self-esteem. Its affirmations and meditations will systematically work to quiet the inner critic and rewire a healthy inner relationship that is nurturing, grounding, empowering and inspiring. A wonderful resource for leaders exploring self-leadership and expanding their own emotional intelligence and relational skill.

~**Amy Elizabeth Fox**
CEO, Mobius Executive Leadership

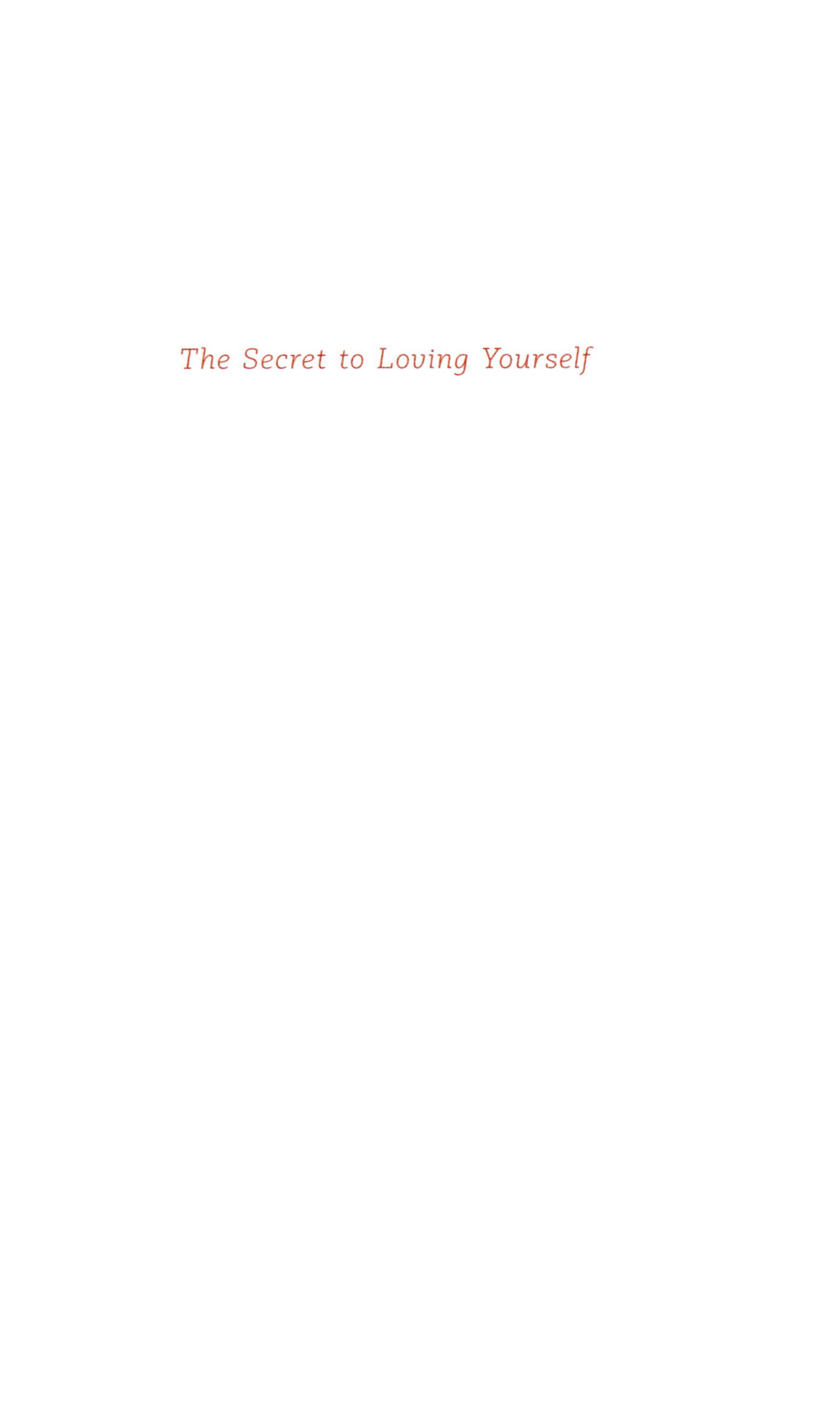

The Secret to Loving Yourself

THE Secret TO LOVING Yourself

Profound Little Messages to Change Your Life

Beth Bardovi, LMFT

Margie Gayle, PsyD

Foreword by Barnet Bain

PRECOCITY PRESS

In memory of Dr. Jack Lee Rosenberg

Jack was a genius and ahead of his time in founding Integrative Body Psychotherapy (IBP). The Good Mother Messages in this book, evolved from his dedication to deepening his love and compassion for himself.

With the blessings of Jack and his wife, Beverly Kitaen Morse, IBP co-developer, we expanded the Messages to help readers embody a deeper love and compassion for themselves.

Jack was our mentor, teacher, and friend. We are forever grateful for his sweetness, fierce spirit and devotion to truth.

Editor: Sara Volle
Creative Director: Susan Shankin
Designer: Barbara Garibay
Photographer: Wieslaw Jarek

ISBN: 978-1-7352921-1-3
Library of Congress Control Number: 2020913114

Published by Precocity Press
Venice, CA 90291

First edition. Printed and bound in the
United States of America

For our children,
Lina, Mo, Matthew & Vanessa.
And for the child inside everyone.

CONTENTS

FOREWORD

OUR WORLD IS CHANGING at warp speed. Things come up that trigger me, that cause me to become reactive, or make me feel anxious, nervous, frightened, or worried. Sometimes it's financial matters, relationship issues, health news, or a deep concern for the wellbeing of loved ones. I have friends going through every one of these challenges right now. I bet you do, too. It is difficult and confronting.

Beth Bardovi and Margie Gayle have been practicing and teaching Integrative Body Psychotherapy for many years. Beth has been my friend and teacher for almost a decade. She helped me realize that most of my troubling thoughts and feelings are the same as, similar to, or familiar in some way to events from my history. Usually my childhood history, boyhood days. Because my body remembers all the long ago hurts, old upsets, old wounds, they can be re-triggered at any time by developments happening now.

The messages in this lovely, beautifully written book are not messages that I received when I was a little boy.

I love you and I give you permission to be who you are.
You can trust your inner voice.
It's not what you do but who you are that I love.

Take that in for a moment . . . how that feels.

If you sense as I do, that uncertainty is the new normal, then reparenting your younger self matters. Lucky for us, *The Secret to Loving Yourself* is a master class in how to go about it.

~**Barnet Bain**
producer of *What Dreams May Come*,
author of *The Book of Doing and Being*

"It has been shown, for instance, that when there are two harps tuned to the same frequency in a room, one a large harp and the other smaller, if a chord is struck in the bigger harp it fills and infuses the little harp with the grandeur and beauty of its resonance and brings it into tuneful harmony. Then, the little harp sounds out its own tune in its own voice. This is one of the unnoticed ways in which a child learns to become herself. Perhaps the most powerful way parents rear children is through the quality of their presence and the atmosphere that pertains in the in-between times of each day. Unconsciously, the child absorbs this and hopefully parents send out enough tuneful spirit for the child to come into harmony with her own voice."

~**John O'Donohue**
from *Beauty, The Invisible Embrace*

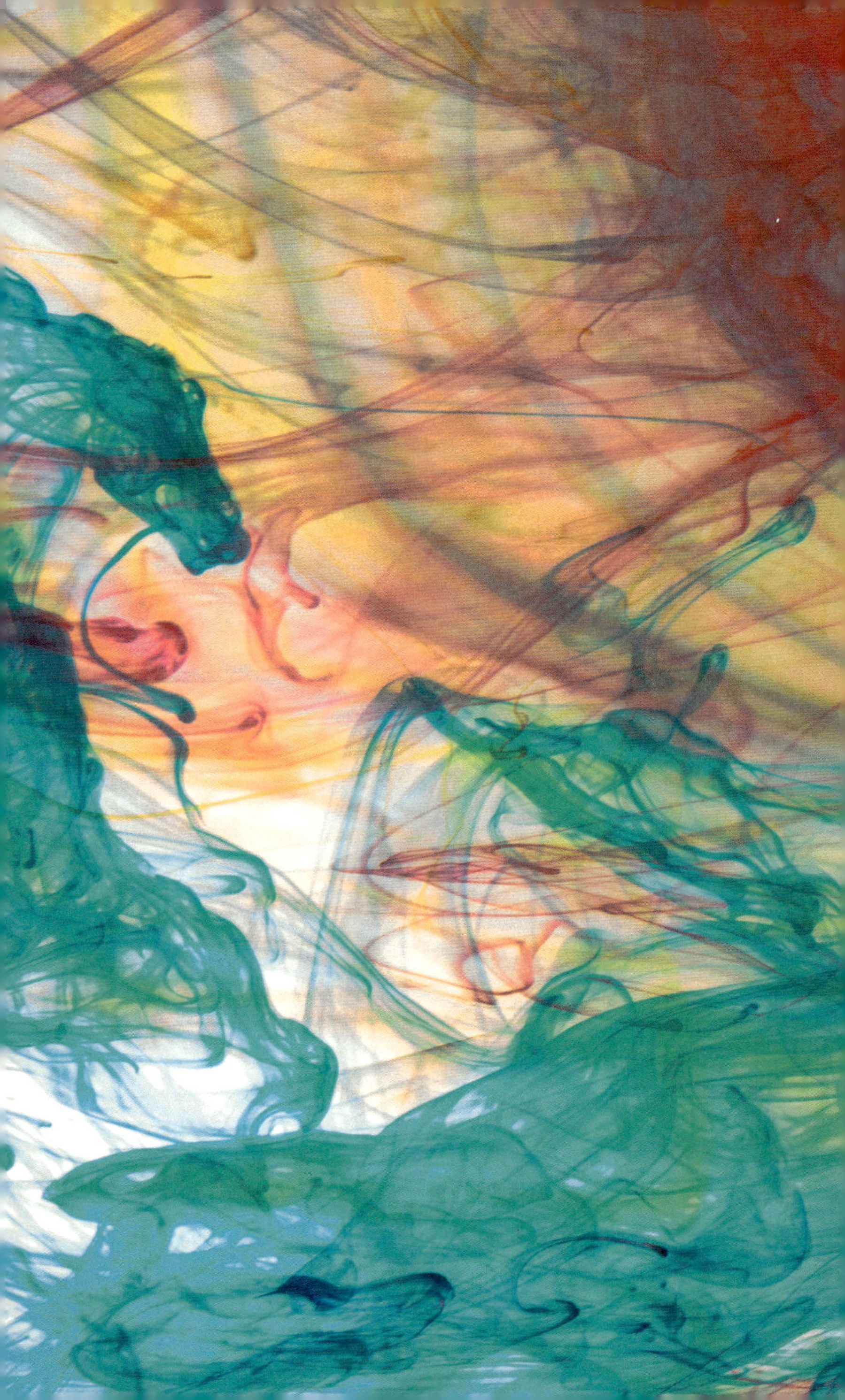

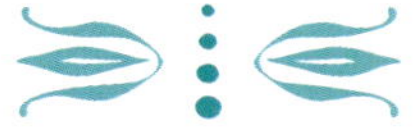

TUNING IN

THIS BOOK IS INTENDED to help you come into harmony with your inner voice and to infuse you with a loving, "tuneful spirit." In our 35 years as psychotherapists, we have witnessed countless clients struggle to find and trust their inner voice. When they discover that quiet, still voice within, they feel loved, understood, and whole.

The secret to loving yourself involves traveling to your inner depths to embrace the child you once were and who remains inside you. Your early experiences develop your emotional blueprint. Today, it's as if there are two voices resounding in your body and mind. One is your adult voice who is integrated and connected to your knowing of who you are. The other voice is your younger self who wasn't always supported and encouraged, and therefore internalized criticism, judgement, and self-doubt. That little voice is activated when you have a triggering emotional experience and you overreact to someone or something. In those moments, you fragment and become that small child trying to manage your adult life.

The truth is that when you're feeling triggered, it's the younger, more vulnerable you who needs to be seen, heard, and comforted by your older, wiser self. These profound, little messages will help you tune in with compassion and visualize your smaller self who is hurting. You can become the soothing parent who scoops up, hugs, and kisses your little one, healing the wounds from your past.

Beginning in infancy, children feel the emotional atmosphere within their family and the quality of their parents' energetic presence. No child experiences perfect parenting, and no one can be a perfect parent. It's impossible for a parent to meet every one of their child's emotional needs.

Most parents learn to parent their children the way they were parented. Parents aren't always able to be emotionally present and in tune with themselves. As a result, they aren't always emotionally present and in tune with their children.

Children absorb the emotional energy of their parents, and look to their parents to know who they are. When the child needs to be filled with the parent's tuneful presence, and the parent is energetically or physically unavailable, the child may feel alone and disconnected. When there is a misattunement, children blame themselves and embody a sense that there must be something wrong with them.

The misattunements and emotional wounds experienced in your early childhood seep into your adult life. They become part of the fabric of your emotional blueprint. This fabric contains the threads of the times you felt known and the thin spots resulting from the times you didn't. It's the thinning in the fabric of your life that contributes to your feelings of fragility. The profound little messages on the following pages are designed to weave in those missing threads, to strengthen you at your core so that your inner life becomes a secure, resilient, and authentic tapestry.

Just as children look to their parents to tell them who they are and to fill their needs, adults often look outside themselves to others to seek validation, reassurance, acceptance, and love. Unconsciously, these early unmet longings are the fragilities adults seek to fill in their significant relationships with lovers and their own children. These longings compel you to try to find that special someone who can see and hear you so that you feel whole. This seeking often leads to disappointment. Just as there are no perfect parents, no partner can meet your every need. Once you reach adulthood only you can fill the emptiness underneath the longing.

Embodying these profound, loving, and tuneful little messages will resonate internally while calming and re-energizing your nervous system and spirit. As you create new patterns of relating with yourself, you begin to heal and build security, trust, and resilience inside. This feeling of well-being as a palpable sensation in your body is what we call constancy. It is in this state of constancy that you faithfully and dependably remain in charge of your emotional life.

At first, these messages might be difficult to take in. Be curious about what is getting in your way. Notice what feelings come up. Chances are your feelings are the same as, similar, or familiar to what you experienced in your family of origin.

It's human nature to gravitate toward what is familiar. That old pull is there because that's how you survived what felt intolerable growing up. However, lasting change requires letting go of old familiar patterns and swimming in uncharted waters. When the adult part of you can step in and be a good parent to your younger self, this early part of you begins to grow and thrive. With this newfound inner support, you learn to swim more skillfully in waters of increasing depth, which allows for transformation and lasting change.

The secret to finding wholeness is to love all of yourself at this core level. As you tune in with compassion and get to know the young child you were, you can be soothed and calmed with understanding. From this practice, you will experience a deeper, richer love for yourself and others. Your important relationships will become based upon love and desire rather than longings and needs. The art of loving someone else begins with the realization that only you can love yourself to wholeness.

Repairing the inner foundation upon which you stand will heal your early emotional wounds and deepen your understanding and compassion for how you first learned to relate to others. From this place of inner stability, you will then relate to yourself and to others differently. Working from the inside allows for deep repair and healing so that your younger self matures to become a coherent, resilient, attuned adult. Being grown up is being at home with yourself. The attuned adult then attunes to their children, their partners and everyone else in their ever widening circle. The secret to loving yourself is to deepen and expand the spaciousness inside so that love is cultivated as a state of being.

PROFOUND LITTLE MESSAGES

These messages are the energetic feeling tones that a parent ideally gives to their child. As we've stated, there is no such thing as a perfect parent. Because of that there are misses in the child feeling tuned into and known by their parents. As the child grows, these misses create gaps in the child's development. These gaps or longings are usually what people come into therapy to fill. Although they don't always have the words for or the knowing, most of their struggles relate back to the gaps and themes in their early development. These themes become the way they dance in relationships, especially intimate ones.

During our sessions with clients, we're listening for and tracking the misses in attunement, emotional injuries, and how they protected themselves when they were young. We are all wired for survival. When triggered, most people revert back to their early coping strategies. So, when you're triggered, it's likely you're responding from where the "miss" was–your early emotional blueprint. If you weren't seen and heard in childhood, and if someone doesn't see and hear you currently, regardless of the significance of the relationship, it's possible you will feel hurt and become fragmented.

This book is intended to help you heal that younger part of yourself, that part of you who becomes activated and can fragment, when the same, similar, or familiar miss in attunement happens. These messages are designed to convey the energetic feeling tone that was either missing or that you didn't get enough of when you were young.

When you feel upset and ask yourself what it is that is triggering you, you're beginning to build your own system of self-attunement. With curiosity, discover how this longing is the same as, similar, or familiar to the hurt feelings you had when you were growing up. What are you seeking or hoping to get from others? Is it to be loved? Wanted? Seen and heard? Understood? Or to feel special?

There are several ways to use this book. To begin, we recommend you find a message that speaks to you. Can you take it in? If you feel soothed and calmed then the next step is to visualize the child who lives inside you and give the message(s) to that them. It's the grownup who gives the message to the child. Who do you see? What did that little child need that they didn't get? How old are they? What is the expression on their face? We encourage you to really get to know them. Then, from a calmed, soothed state, re-read the messages to your younger self.

We suggest you slow down. Take your time as you read the verses. They impart the energetic feeling tone that an ideal parent would give to their child. Let the energy of these messages wash through you.

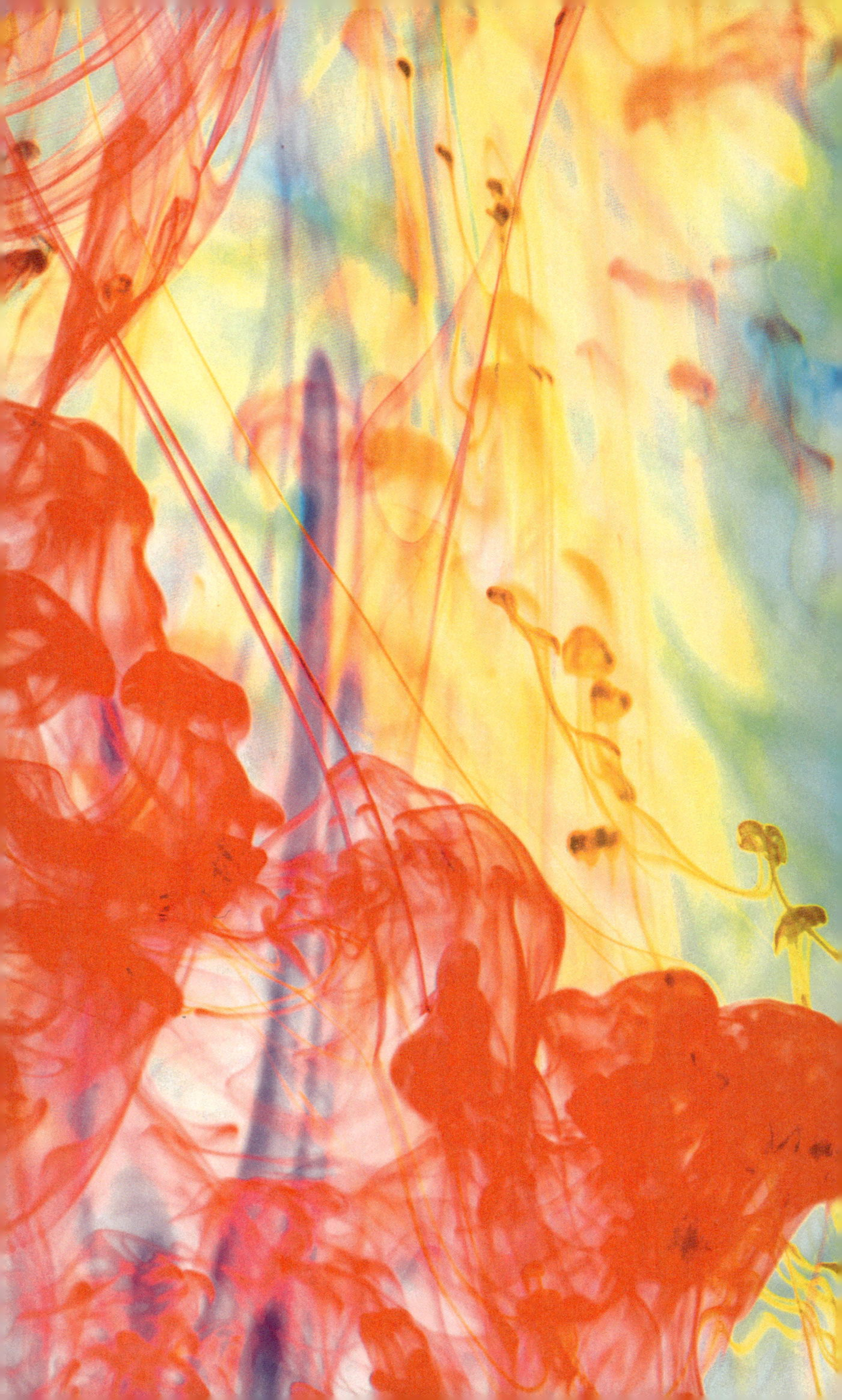

I **love you.**

No matter what, I love you.
I thrill at the sight of you.
I find you irresistible.
Love is in that special look we share.
Love is how we know each other.
In knowing you I soften.
I feel your tender heart.
Our love is for always, my love for
you and your love for me.

I love you.

I want you.

I choose you.

I celebrate you.

I tingle all over when I see you.

I embrace you.

You are a gift to me.

I want you.

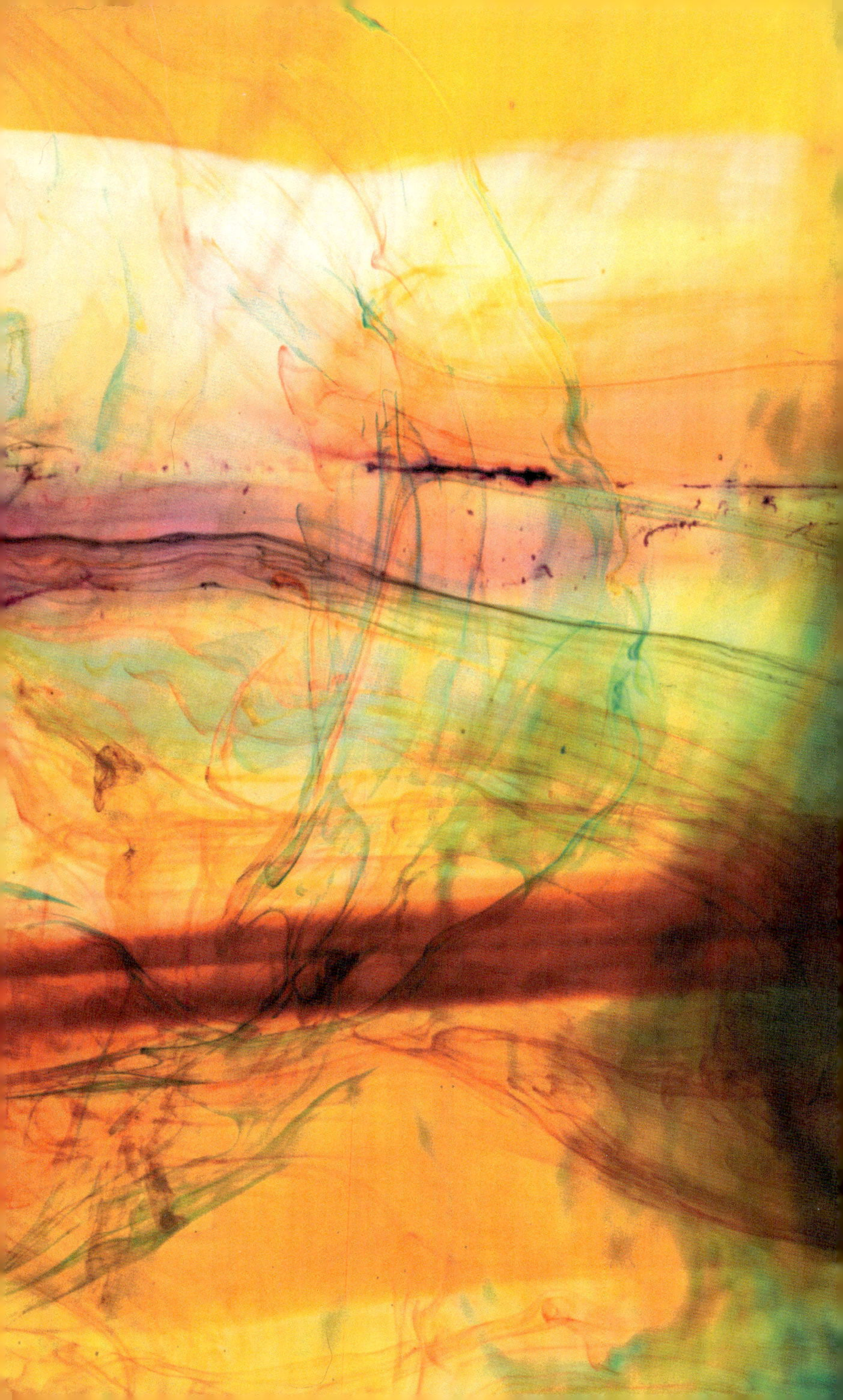

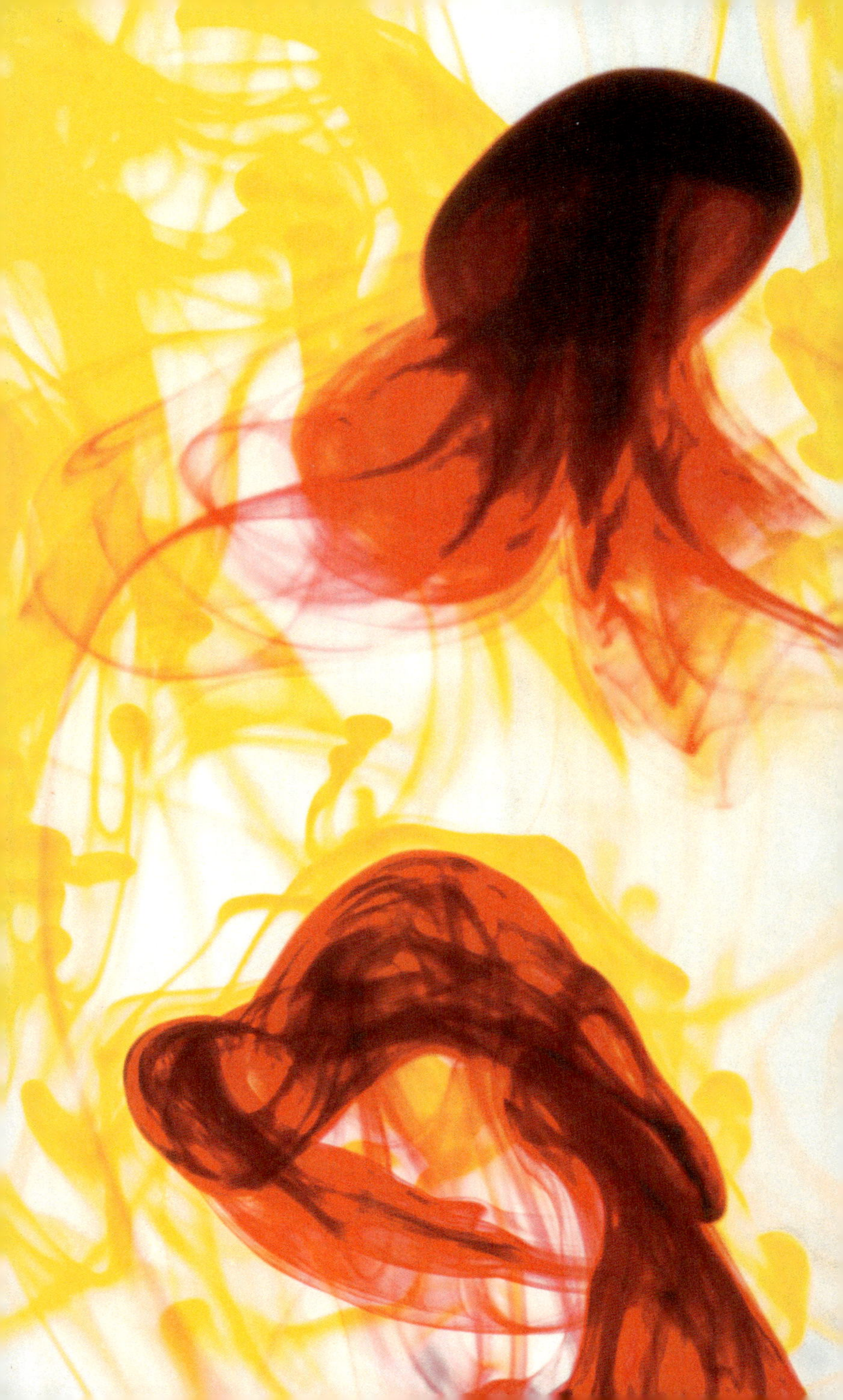

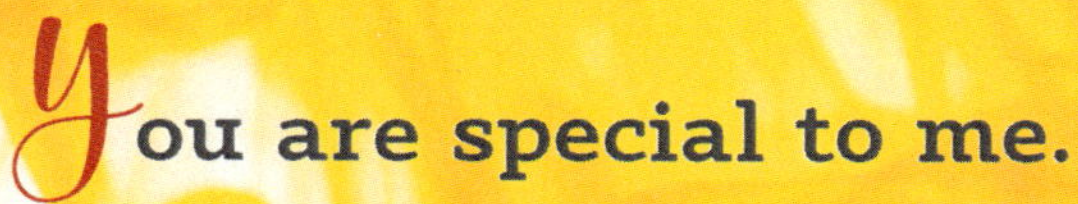

You are special to me.

There's no one else like you.

I adore you.

You are a blessing in my life—so endearing, so beautiful, so precious.

I delight in you.

You are special to me.

I see you and I hear you.

I am present with you.
I sit with you in what is.
I tune into how you feel.
I know when you need comforting
and I know when you need space.
I see you and
I hear you with clarity.

I see you and I hear you.

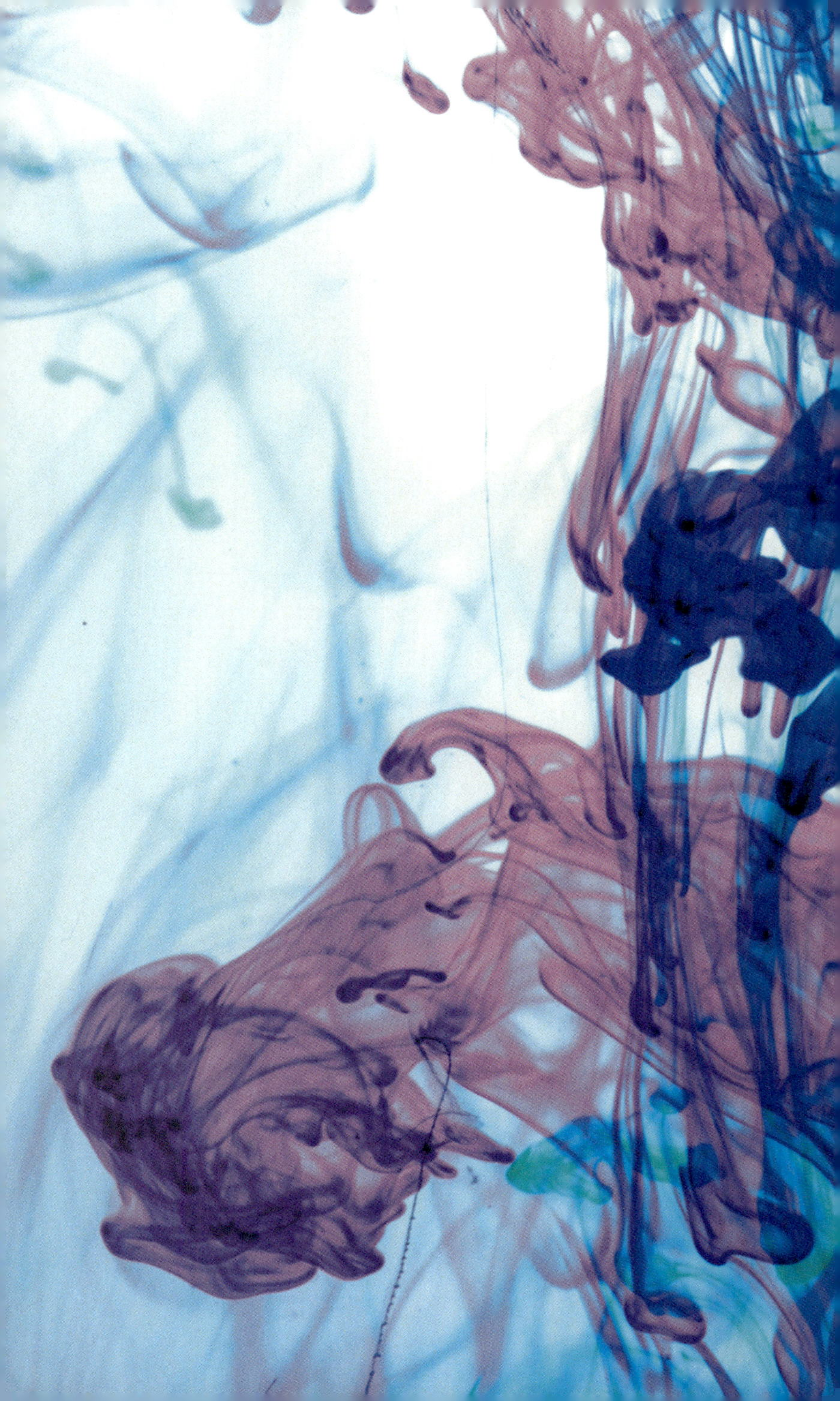

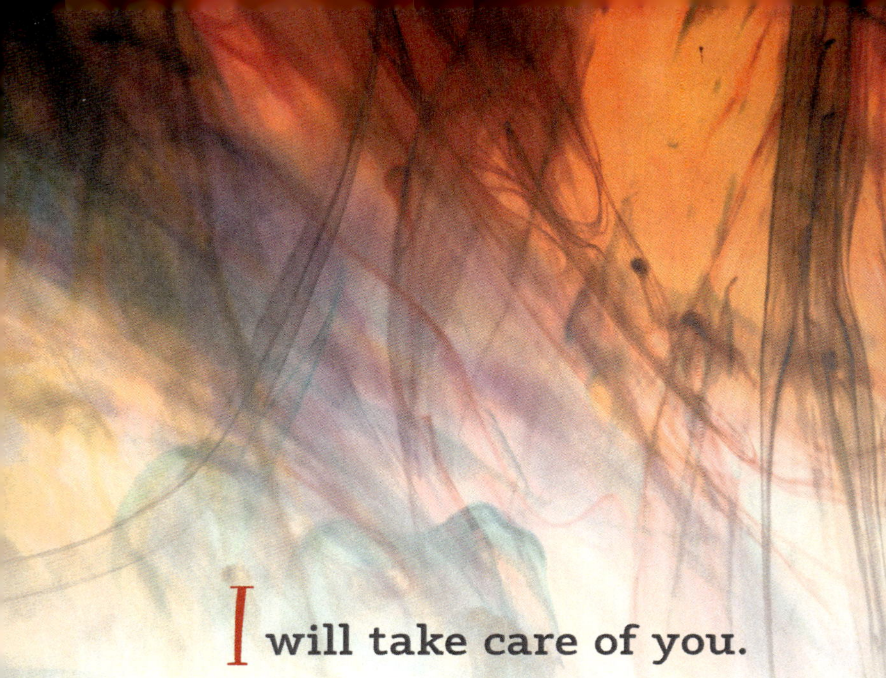

I will take care of you.

I will hold you in my arms.

I will protect you and keep you safe.

If you fall down,

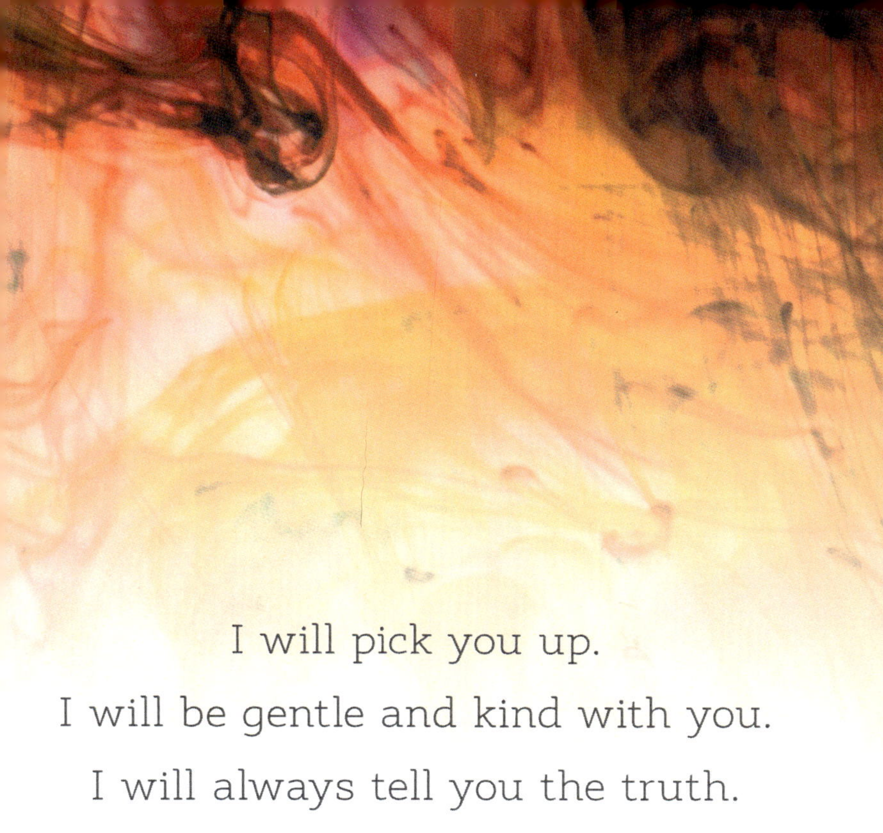

I will pick you up.

I will be gentle and kind with you.

I will always tell you the truth.

I will take care of you.

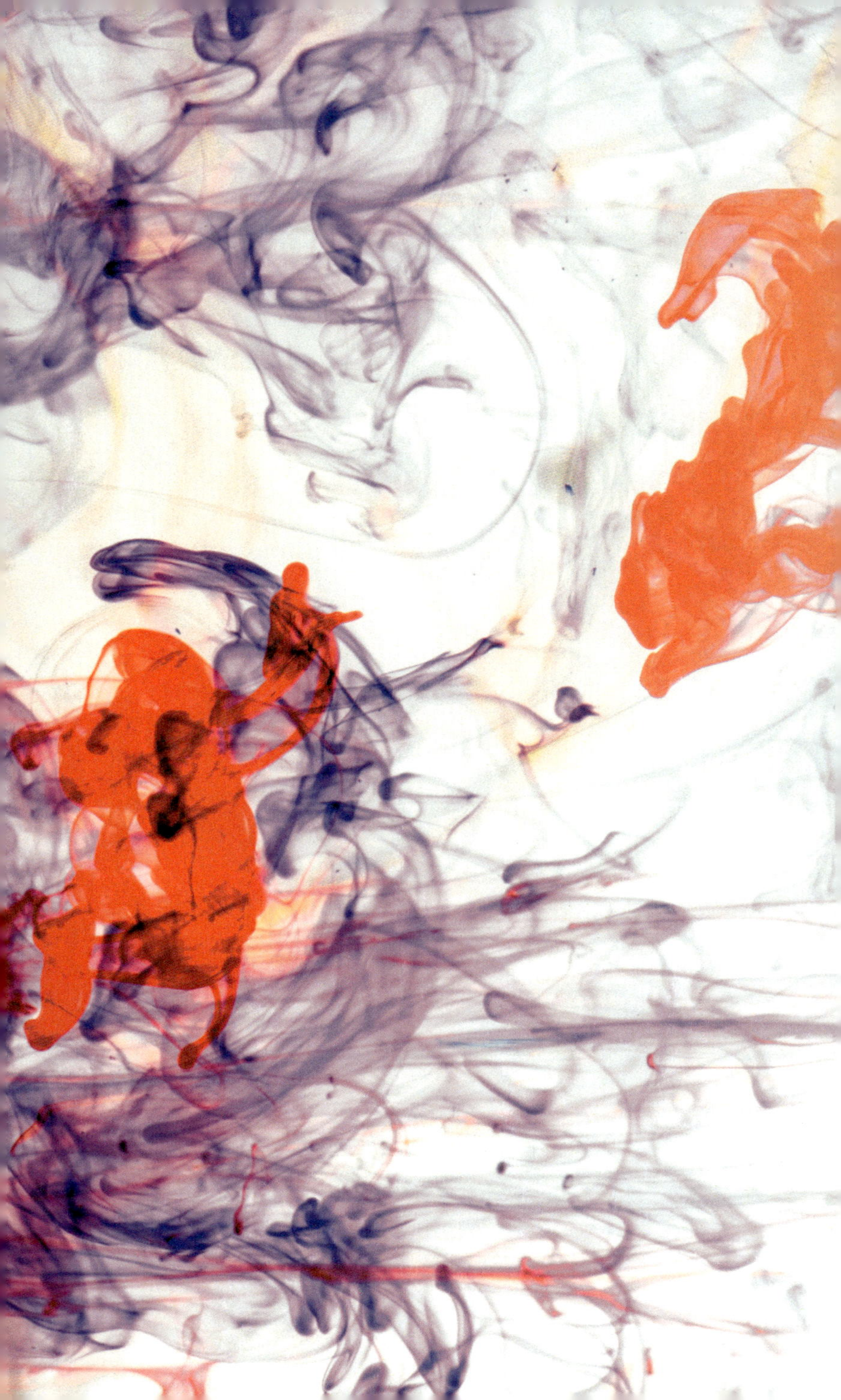

I will always be here for you.

I will support you and
stand up for you.
If you feel lost, I will help you find
your way back.
I will not abandon you.
If you need me I am here.

I will always be here for you.

My love will make you well.

I know when you're not well and
I will take care of you.
I will encourage you to rest.
I will comfort you.
I will pay attention to you.
I will treat you with tenderness.

My love will make you well.

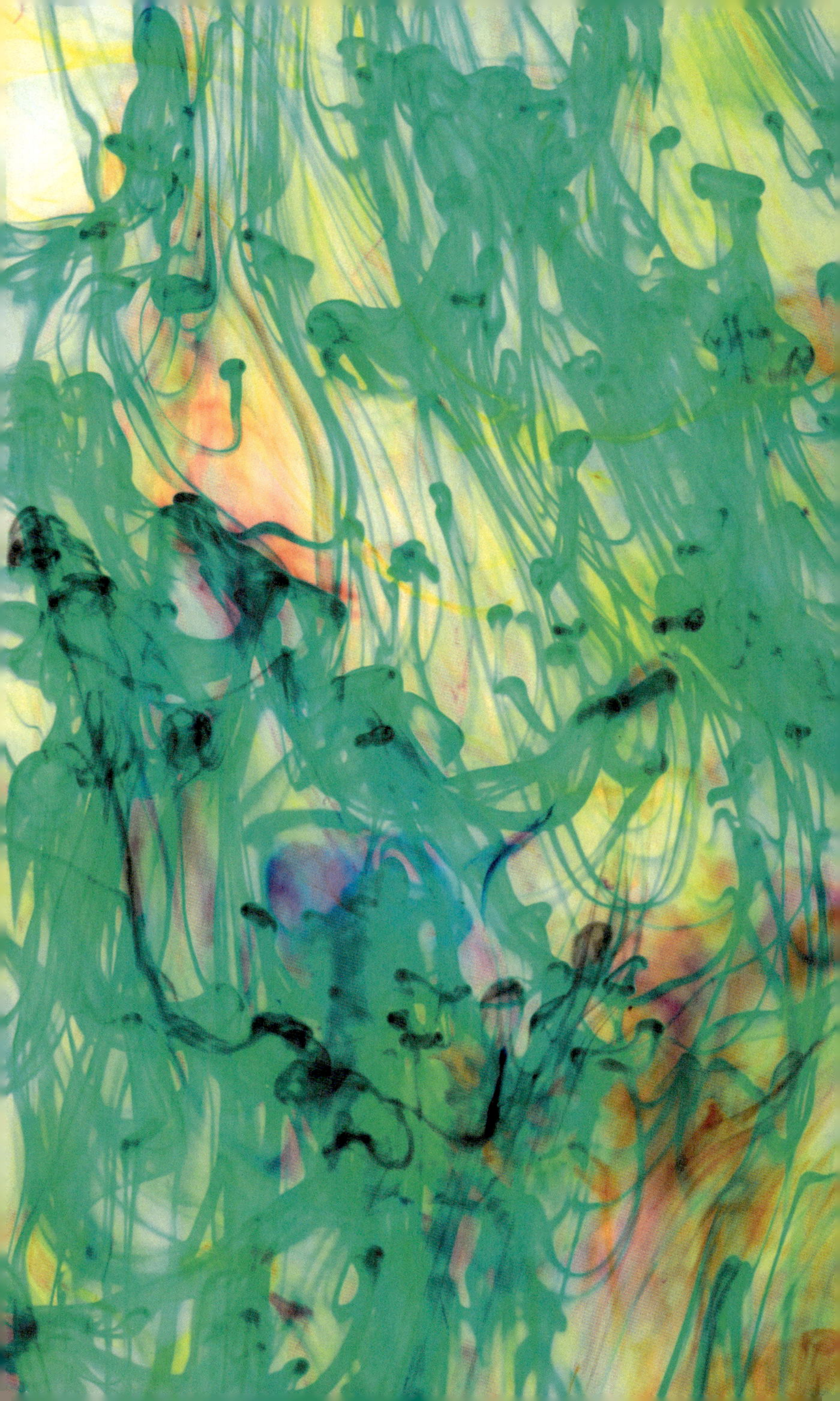

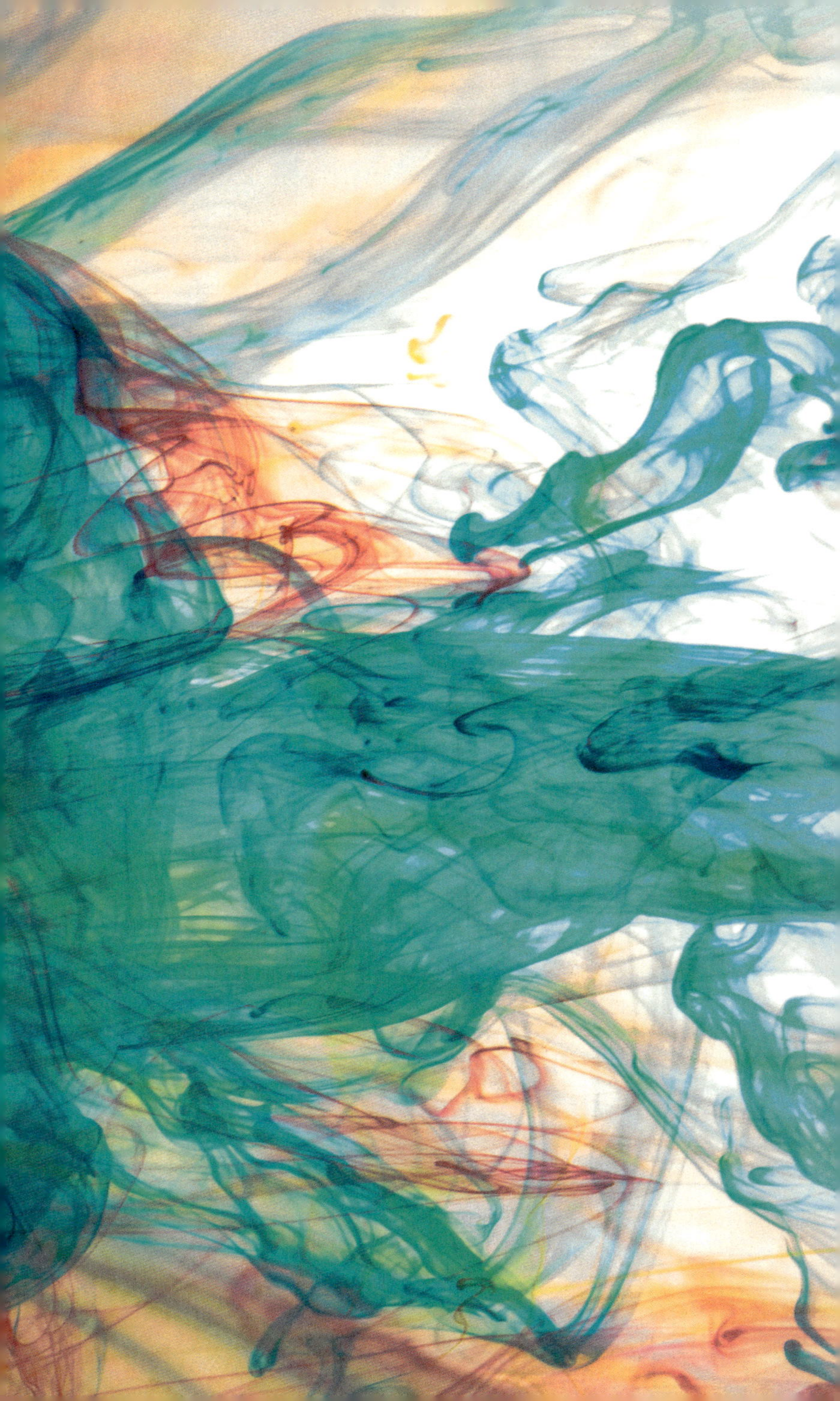

Sometimes I will tell you no,
and that's because I love you.

Because I love you,
I will protect you.
I will alert you if you're
about to harm yourself.
I will urge you to pause so that
you act in your best interest.

Sometimes I will tell you no,
and that's because I love you.

I love you and I give you permission to be who you are.

I believe in you.
Radiate in your own light.
Embrace your essence.

Express your spirit.
You shine when grounded,
present, and connected.

I love you and I give you permission to be who you are.

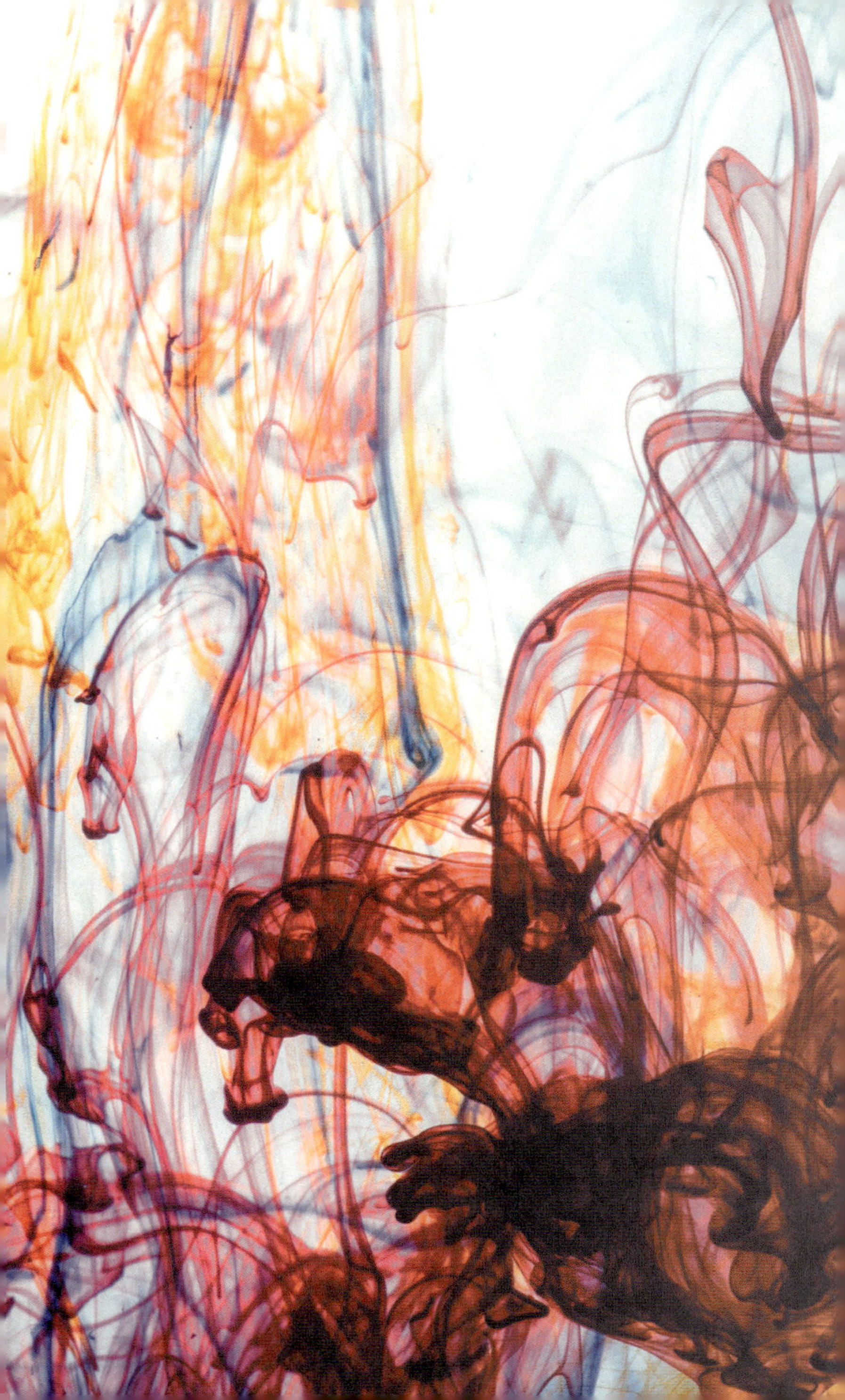

It is not what you do,
it is who you are that I love.

I treasure your spirit.
You are a most precious being.
You are special and uniquely you.
I honor your rhythm.
I bask in your essence.
When you are you,
you are beautiful.

It is not what you do,
it is who you are that I love.

You don't have to be afraid anymore.

I am here and will keep you safe.
Together, we'll acknowledge your fear.
I will help you understand and explore what is scaring you.
Together we can face anything.

You don't have to be afraid anymore.

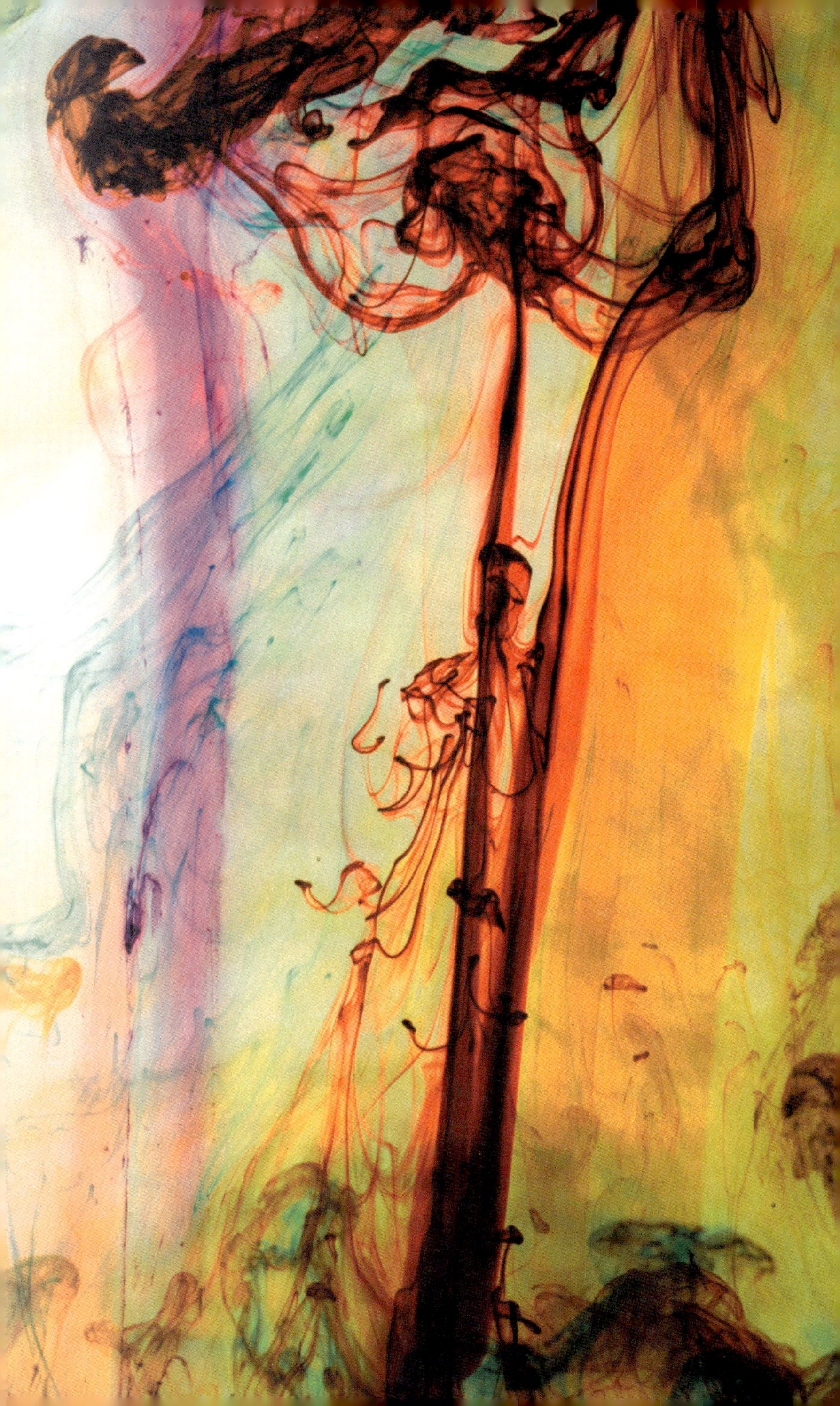

You don't have to be alone anymore.

Find me. I am always with you. Breathe—breathe as if you're breathing for the first time.

Breathe to discover the bridge
that connects me to you.
In the stillness inside,
know I am always here.

**You don't have to be
alone anymore.**

You can trust your inner voice.

It's your voice inside that knows.
Drop into silence.
Listen with intention.
Deepen the witness and
stand in your truth.
Your truth is your wisdom.
Your wisdom is your truth.

You can trust your inner voice.

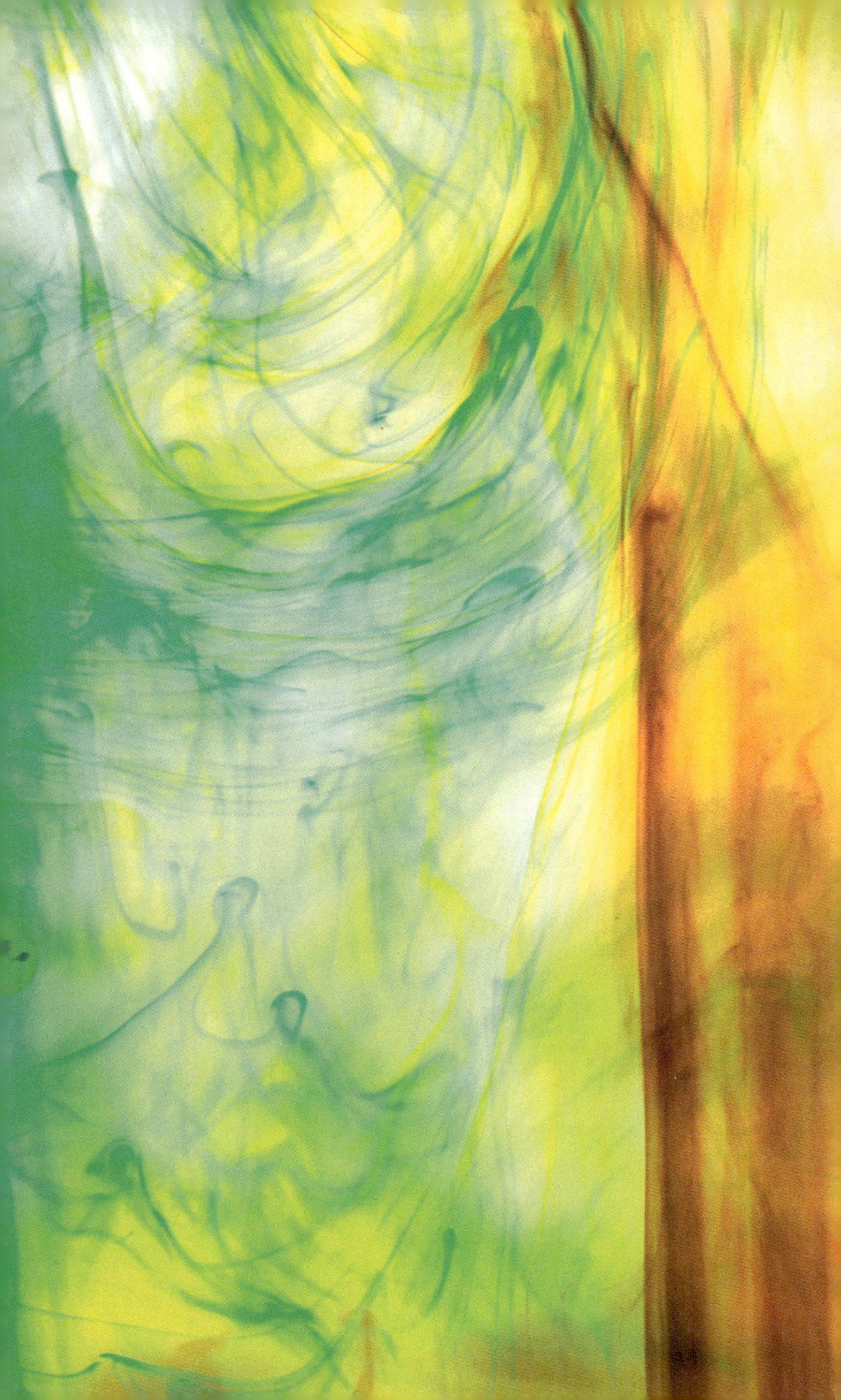

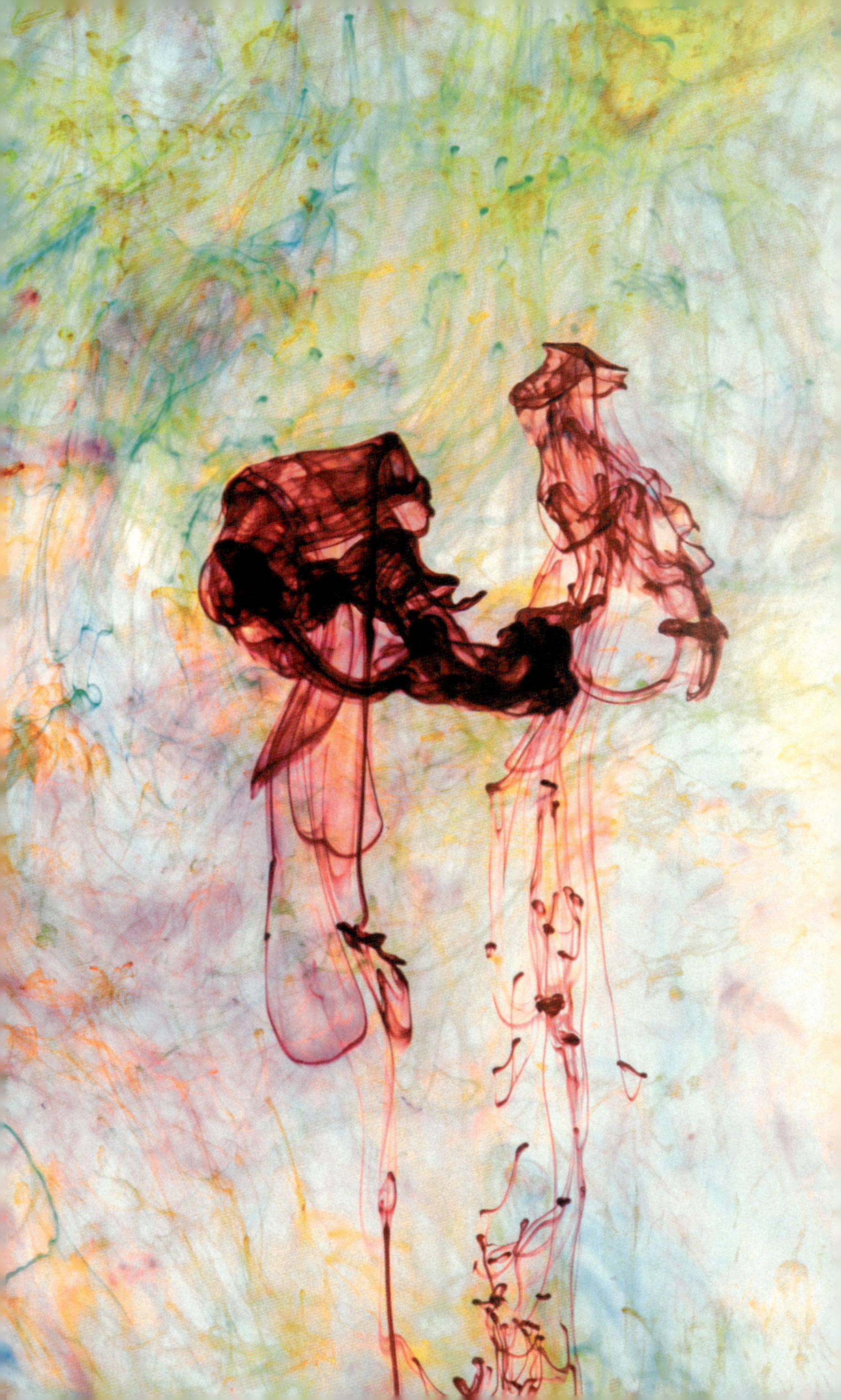

You can trust me.

I listen to you with curiosity
and acceptance.
My desire is to know you deeply.
Sometimes it's not easy to say
what's true.
Even with the most difficult truths
you will not lose me.

You can trust me.

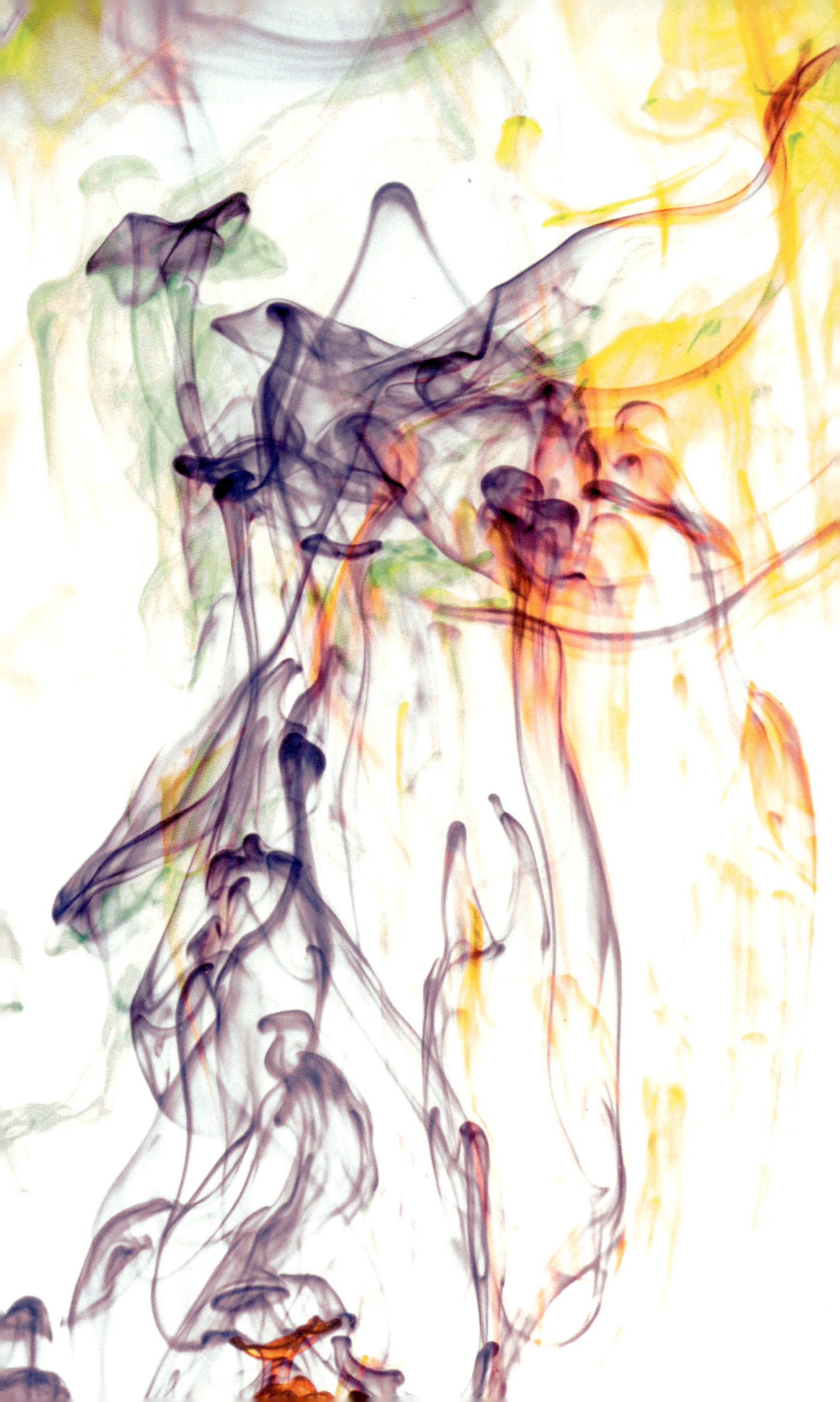

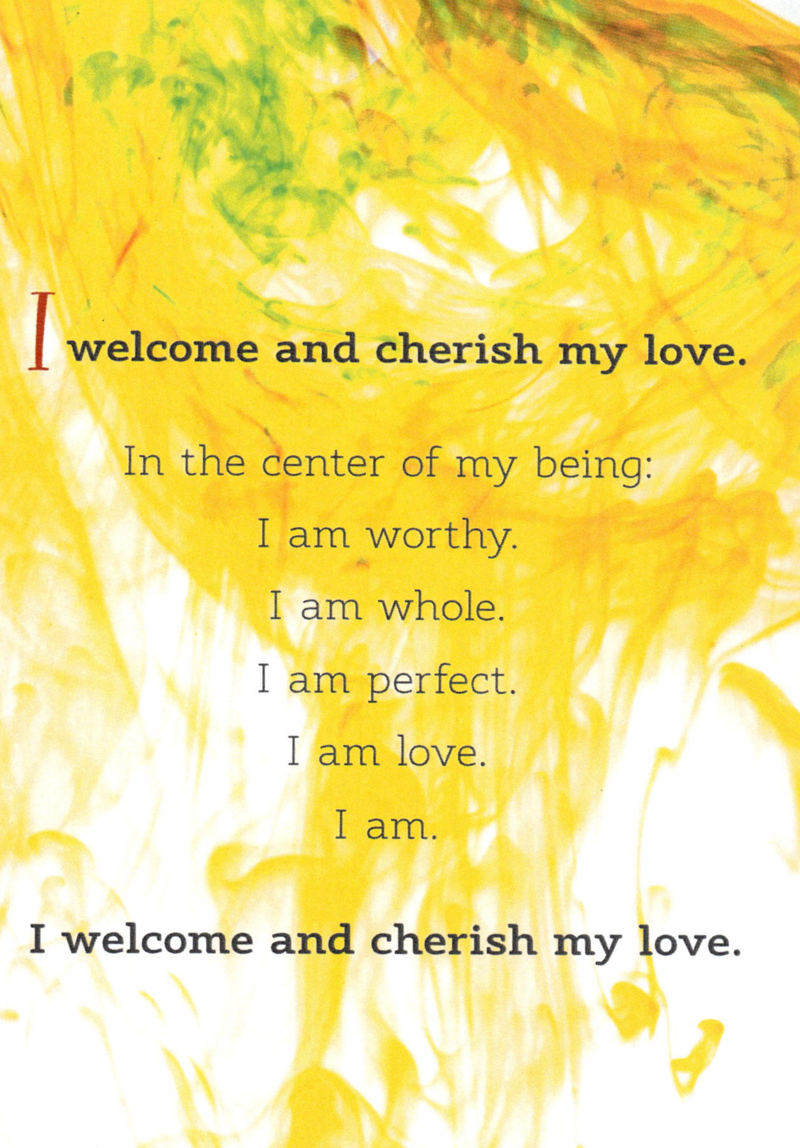

I welcome and cherish my love.

In the center of my being:

I am worthy.

I am whole.

I am perfect.

I am love.

I am.

I welcome and cherish my love.

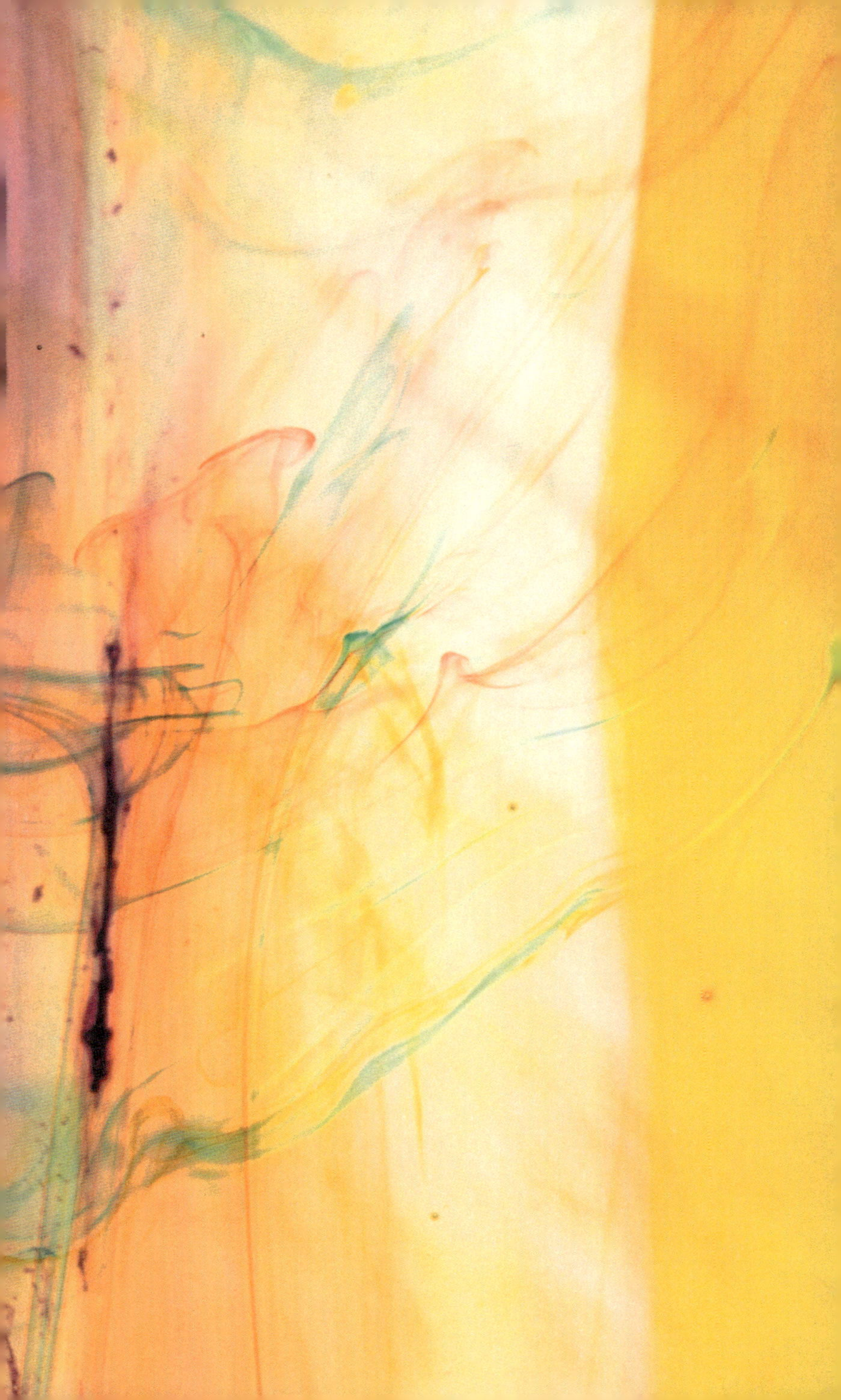

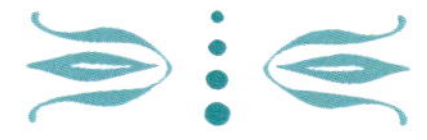

DEVELOPING SELF-ATTUNEMENT

IT'S IMPERATIVE THAT the adult part of you builds a relationship with your inner child based upon trust and authenticity. It's important to give these messages to your younger self every day. When you consistently convey these messages, the young child in you will learn to trust that you will show up for them when you say you will. Your inner child will know that you will follow through and do what you say. Do your words and behaviors match? Just as with any relationship, it's one of the ways we look to see if someone is trustworthy.

All children have tender hearts. Having the courage to honor this tenderness and vulnerability that lives inside you promotes deep and profound healing of your sensitivities and shame. If you make that commitment to honoring who you are, your inner child will feel felt and known by you. You will build and enjoy a more resilient life and be less easily triggered. This makes you stronger, and then it's easier to state your truth until it becomes second nature and you embody who you truly are—your authentic self.

JOURNAL PRACTICES

A regular physical exercise practice maintains your health, strength, and flexibility. Similarly, you can develop your emotional "muscle" so that you become more constant in your sense of wellbeing, stability, and resilience. Practice embodying these profound little messages. Use them whenever you want to soothe, calm, and connect inside. They're wonderful to recite at night as you relax and fall asleep.

First Practice

Memorize these fifteen messages by reading them often and noticing which ones soothe you in moments when you feel triggered.

I love you.

I want you.

You are special to me.

I see you and I hear you.

I will take care of you.

I will always be here for you.

My love will make you well.

Sometimes I will tell you no,
and that's because I love you.

I love you and I give you permission to be who you are.

It is not what you do, it is who you are that I love.

You don't have to be afraid anymore.

You don't have to be alone anymore.

You can trust me.

You can trust your inner voice.

I welcome and cherish my love.

Second Practice

From memory, write the messages on a page in your journal. Draw a line under the last message you remember.

Look back at the list of all fifteen messages. Then, under the line you've drawn, write the messages you couldn't remember.

Repeat this for 30 days. After 30 days look and see if there is a pattern to the messages you wrote under the line. Often the messages you've forgotten are the ones that you didn't get enough of when you were young.

Third Practice

One at a time, write each message and personalize what this message means to you. For example, write "I love you" at the top of the page, then put your pen down.

Take 10 big breaths through your mouth, high up into your chest.

Visualize and imagine yourself as a child. Trust whatever image you see. It can be a memory or from a photograph. Who do you see? How old are you? What is the expression on your face? What are you wearing? Where are you?

Now bring the adult part of you into the scene. Feel into what this child inside needs and impart this feeling tone authentically and energetically. With meaning, tell your younger self, "I love you." Take a slow deep breath. It's best to repeat this a few times.

Observe what comes up for you in that experience. What does the child part of you feel? What does the adult part of you feel? Write it in your journal.

Ask yourself what this feeling tone means for you. For example, someone might feel special. Someone else might feel known and supported. This is how you personalize what this message means to you.

Do this for each message. Go in order, don't skip one if it doesn't immediately resonate for you.

Again, it may be one of the messages you didn't receive enough when you were young.

PRESENCE, CENTERING, AND GROUNDING PRACTICES

When you get triggered and fragment, it's because an old theme that is similar to something you experienced in your family of origin is felt in the present. When fragmented as an adult, it feels like an over-reaction to the current event. You have fallen out of coherence and you are not in harmony with yourself. These emotions feel overwhelming today because they were too much or too intense for you to have as a child.

Infants and small children do not have the ability to self regulate or to self soothe. They depend on their parents for this. Humans are relational beings and children innately know when they want closeness and connection. Children can feel when they have needs or are in distress. When they want closeness, they gaze into their parent's eyes. If their mother or father responds with connection they feel filled up. If they have a need or are in discomfort they cry to alert their parents to attend to them. If their need is met they calm and relax.

Remember, it's impossible to meet an infant or small child's needs 100% of the time. Their earliest form of self protection when their needs are not met is to split off or space out to avoid feeling what is intolerable. Unless it is brought to awareness, this early, unconscious, automatic coping strategy of spacing out continues into adulthood and throughout life. When you are split off or spaced out, you are in the past and you are not present. When you are not present, you are not grounded. Splitting off can feel like you are shut down, unbalanced, or a bit foggy.

Being present means that you are open, accepting, and receptive to what is happening as it is happening. It is a state of curiosity and wonder rather than one of expectation.

When fully present most adults have the capacity to tolerate their emotions. Noticing when you are split off and having a practice to get yourself back to the present moment is powerful. Developing this deeper form of mindfulness allows you to be in charge of living a more fulfilled and connected life.

The following practices are quick and easy ways to get yourself present, grounded, and centered.

Presence Practice

To become present: Snap your fingers rapidly, look around the room and say out loud the colors and objects you see. Try doing this as quickly as possible to the rhythm of your snapping fingers.

For example, "gray cat, pink flower, black pants, purple blanket, blue bowl," etc.

When it becomes easy for you to name the colors and the objects, you are present. When you are split off, this practice is difficult to do.

If you find yourself splitting off while with others, you can bring yourself back to presence by silently naming colors and objects.

Centering & Grounding Practice

To find your grounding: Stand in your bare feet, with your knees slightly bent.

Spread and widen your toes and place them firmly on the floor.

Gently rock your weight back and forth and from side to side.

Stand with slightly more weight centered in the balls of your feet than your heels.

Spread your toes again and replant them on the floor creating a landing pad so your weight is evenly distributed across the width of your foot.

Find your balance.

Place one hand just below your belly button. Take a few slow, deep breaths through your nose into your hand, and let your feet sink into the floor.

You will feel centered and grounded.

BREATHING PRACTICES

Breathing is connected to your early development and is a way to return to contact and intimacy with yourself. During misattunements in your childhood, you may have learned to cut off by holding or inhibiting your breathing to protect yourself from emotions that felt too intense. This cutting off can create chronic holding patterns in your body. These holding patterns can manifest in many ways, including a clenched jaw, a tightening in your chest, chronic back pain, or a tense feeling of carrying the weight of the world on your shoulders.

Remember, when you are triggered and fragmented it is the young child who is activated. When you feel triggered and you take a few deep breaths, the old holding patterns are interrupted. Breathing can be a bridge to reconnect your adult self with your younger self. Breathing is a way of taking charge of your internal state of being. Different ways of breathing engage the two parts of the autonomic nervous system—the sympathetic and parasympathetic nervous systems. It's important to know when you need to calm and soothe yourself (parasympathetic) and when you need more energy and vitality (sympathetic). Essentially, when you feel present, connected, and grounded, your nervous system is in balance and you feel calm and alert.

When you are triggered or upset, your nervous system is out of balance, and you feel fragmented.

Your brain is the command center for your nervous system. Brain scans show that when you're triggered, the survival part of your brain, your amygdala, lights up. When your amygdala is firing, your prefrontal cortex, the reasoning and higher thinking part of your brain, goes offline. Conscious, deep breathing serves to rebalance your nervous system by calming your amygdala, and reactivating your prefrontal cortex. When your amygdala is calm and your prefrontal cortex is functioning you are able to think and act in a clearer, more grounded, and authentic manner.

The following breathing practices are designed to help you balance your nervous system. From a more balanced state, you can access the adult part of you so that you can relate to your younger self differently. This is a way to develop more resilience. Increased resilience allows you to stay in contact and intimacy with yourself and to quickly recover when you are fragmented.

For Calming, Soothing, and Engaging Your Parasympathetic Nervous System

All breaths in this section are in and out through your nose.

To foster self-attunement (the ability to tune in and know yourself): Put one hand on your chest and the other hand on your belly and take slow deep breaths through your nose.

Your exhale needs to be twice as long as your inhale. These slow deep breaths with the exhale longer than your inhale engage your parasympathetic nervous system and enable you to relax.

In this calm, attuned state take time to check in with your inner child. From this state of being you have the best chance of seeing, understanding, and listening to what that little child inside of you needs.

To alleviate anxiety: This breathing practice helps reduce anxiety because it gives your brain something to focus on other than your anxious thoughts. Count your breaths in and out. Remember, all breaths in this sequence are through your nose, both inhale and exhale.

Inhale for a count of four into your belly. Expand your belly out on the inhale. Do not exhale and continue inhaling into your upper chest for a count of four.

Hold your breath for a count of four.

Exhale for a count of eight. Toward the end of your exhale contract your belly in. It is helpful when breathing into your belly to place your hand on it. When you breathe into your chest, place your hand there.

Repeat this for five to ten rounds. After completing five to ten rounds, breathe naturally, close your eyes and notice what you feel in your body.

Inhale into Belly

1 - 2 - 3 - 4

Inhale into Chest

1 - 2 - 3 - 4

Hold your breath

1 - 2 - 3 - 4

Exhale slowly

1 - 2 - 3 - 4 - 5 - 6 - 7 - 8

For Building Energy and Engaging Your Sympathetic Nervous System

All breaths in this section are in and out through your mouth.

Start by sitting or laying down. This will allow you to build energy and contain it. To find grounding, place your feet flat on the floor with more weight in the balls of your feet. This is where you both root and rebound.

To wake your body up and increase your sense of aliveness: Take five to ten big breaths through your mouth into your upper chest. Keep your breath soft on the exhale. Do not push it out. When you've completed this set, take a slow breath in through your nose.

Check in. What do you feel in your body? You might begin to notice some tingling or sensations. This is your body waking up and getting energized. It's natural if you feel light-headed or a bit dizzy. Use the presence practice on page 44 to ground the energy in your body. This will take away the dizziness or light-headedness.

Repeat this several times. The more you do it the more comfortable you will become with it and you will be able to increase the number of breaths you take.

To wake your body up and increase your sense of aliveness with an emphasis on opening your chest: Bring your hands into a prayer pose and turn your finger tips in so they are touching your chest. Bring your elbows up to shoulder height.

With your hands in this position take five to ten big breaths through your mouth into your upper chest, pushing your palms together on the exhale. This creates an isometric sensation. By stressing your muscles this way it allows a holding pattern to release. Initially your chest will tighten. Ideally your chest will open when you complete the breathing cycle.

When you have completed this set, take a slow breath in through your nose.

Check in. What do you feel in your body?

Repeat this process several times. The more you do it the more comfortable you will become with it. With time you will be able to increase how many breaths you take.

To build energy and help spread it through your body: This practice involves taking a double inhale. First, bring the air to your lower lungs then right away, take another inhale and fill your upper chest.

Exhale slowly and softly. It's in the slow exhale that your body relaxes and allows your energy to spread through you. Take five to ten breaths.

When you have completed this set, take a slow breath in through your nose.

Check in. What do you feel in your body?

Repeat this process several times. Remember, the more you do it the more comfortable you will become with it and you will be able to increase the number of breaths you take.

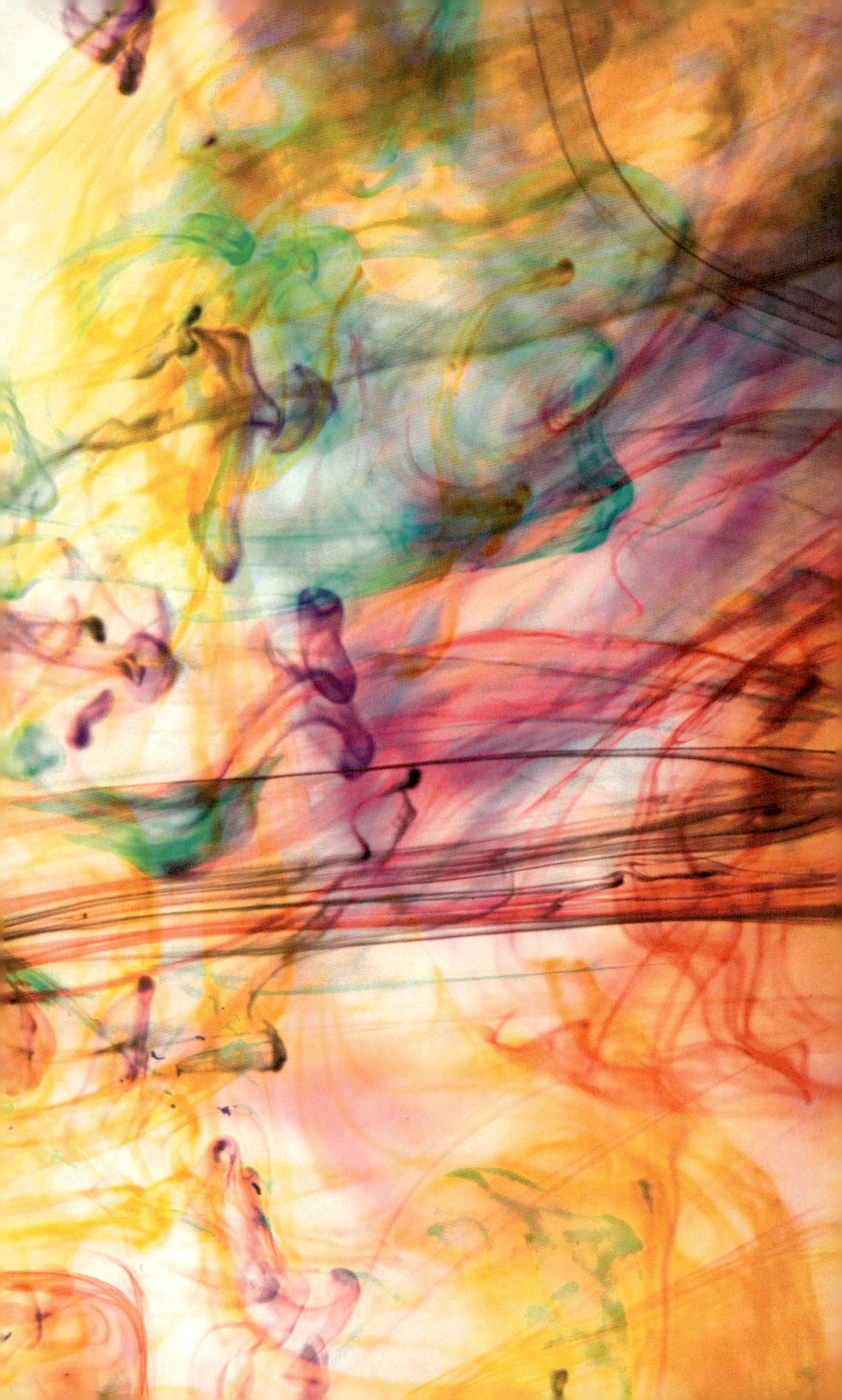

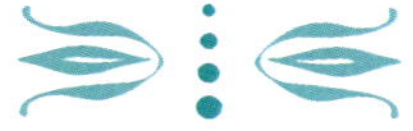

EMBODYING A TUNEFUL SPIRIT

THE INFORMATION AND practices in this book will help you heal the younger part of yourself. To achieve lasting and transformational growth, you need to let go of old and familiar ways that no longer serve you. Deep repair and healing takes place when the adult part of you and the younger part of you can build a mutual relationship based upon trust, understanding, and authenticity.

Creating these new patterns of relating with yourself builds coherence, security, resilience, and well-being as a palpable feeling in your body. When you feel well in your being, you are connected to your inner wisdom, your serenity, and your joy. Your internal state is balanced as you cultivate attunement and intimacy with yourself. As your knowing of yourself deepens, your relationships with others will grow and become more harmonious.

Love lives inside you. The secret to loving yourself is to be fully present. When you're open, accepting, curious, receptive, and responsive to what is happening inside, you are loving yourself at your deepest level.

ACKNOWLEDGMENTS

Humans are relational beings and grow in connection with others. We would like to acknowledge and thank the following people who have influenced, supported, encouraged, and guided us in writing this book:

Jack Lee Rosenberg, DDS, PhD, visionary, founder of Integrative Body Psychotherapy, and originator of the Good Mother Messages, and Beverly Kitaen Morse, PhD, co-developer of Integrative Body Psychotherapy—our mentors, teachers, and friends. We are deeply grateful for all of the gifts we have received from you.

Barney Saltzberg, for your friendship and for all of your encouragement, support and mentoring of us and for helping us bring this book to fruition.

Susan Strick, for your friendship, sharing motherhood and all your legal help and advice along the way.

Riley Smith, MA, LMFT, IBP practitioner, colleague, and friend. Our heartfelt gratitude for guiding us to Susan Shankin.

Susan Shankin, book designer and publisher. We are grateful to you for your artistry and for adding the color. Without you, we couldn't have birthed this book.

Sara Volle, our editor. Thank you for your excellent refinements.

Our clients and our global IBP community, who have influenced us with their courage to look inside and do their deep work. It's our privilege and honor to be a part of your journey.

Carlos Platon Tornes, III, for your sweetness, love, and constancy, your devotion to yours, mine, and others' creativity, and your steady guidance and encouragement of my work and this book.

Gary Bardovi, the love of my life, and whose love, constant support, and belief in me is a rare and precious gift.

Lina and Mo Bardovi, you've both taught me new levels of love and loving. You inspire me to be the best Mom I can be. So proud of who each of you are. Lina, I love you more than all the stars in the sky. Mo, I love you more than all the grains of sand in the world.

Vin Fichter, for your good heart, and for being the father of Matthew and Vanessa.

Matthew and Vanessa Fichter, you are my greatest loves. You've gifted me with your gentle hearts and fierce spirits.

ABOUT THE AUTHORS

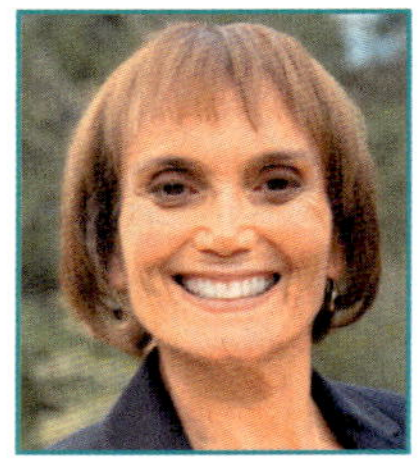

BETH BARDOVI, MA, LMFT has been a Licensed Marriage & Family Therapist in Santa Monica, CA since 1985. She has taught Integrative Body Psychotherapy (IBP) in the United States, Canada and Europe beginning in 1989. She is an IBP practitioner and IBP teacher. Beth served as Director of the Los Angeles Central IBP Institute, and is the Co-Founder and Executive Director of the IBP Institute in Italy.

Beth is a Transformational Faculty member of Mobius Executive Leadership and works with CEO's and business leaders of Fortune 500 Companies.

Her goal is to tap into the innate wisdom of body, mind, and spirit to liberate human potential. She uses breath to balance the nervous system, to change and release old habitual holding patterns, and to allow a deeper more authentic experience of self. Beth believes well-being is a body experience that increases joy, resilience, and aliveness and leads to deep and lasting transformation.

bethbardovi.com

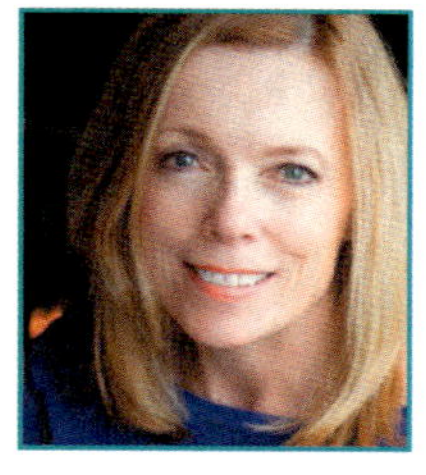

Margie Gayle, PsyD is a licensed psychologist in California, a Registered Professional Counselor (RPC) in Canada, and a Registered Clinical Counselor (RCC) in British Columbia, Canada. The Los Angeles Central Institute of Integrative Body Psychotherapy (IBP) certified her as an IBP practitioner in 2008 and as an IBP teacher in 2014.

Margie now directs the IBP BC Institute and operates a private IBP practice in Vancouver, British Columbia. In Spring, 2020, she launched "The Core Self Transformation," an online educational program designed to introduce the general public to IBP's transformational personal growth work.

Her goals are to help her students and clients develop a deeper sense of self-awareness of their body-mind connection; expand their capacity for emotional depth and authenticity; discover powerful methods to remain present, grounded, and centered; and experience a sense of wholeness and connection inside, so that they feel empowered and in charge of their lives.

margiegayle.com

Made in the USA
Las Vegas, NV
02 May 2021

22332908R00045